Alkaline Herbal Therapy:

15 Tutorials How To Combine And Use Medicinal Herbs To Heal Illnesses Without Pills

Table of content

Introduction

You will almost certainly have heard the concerns which have been echoing around the medical world for the last few years. The biggest one of these is the worry that traditional drugs, such as penicillin and antibiotics are no longer able to treat all diseases. These types of drugs have been the fail safe for the medical industry for years. However, there are now an increasing number of cases where antibiotics and similar modern medicines are having no effect on specific bacteria. It is a matter of grave concern that these bacteria have evolved to become immune to the antibiotics.

The solution may seem surprising but there are an increasing number of studies being done into the effectiveness of herbal medicine; in particular alkaline herbal medicine. In many ways this is a perfectly rational way of dealing with disease; herbs are natural and, by using them, you are engaging with natural and allowing the body to heal itself. However, there are many people who look to exploit the herbal industry. In general the regulations are looser; there is more room for unscrupulous traders to sell alkaline herbs which are not what they say they are or will not help your condition. This is why it is essential to know some of the more popular herbs and confirm what they can or cannot do; it is the best way to avoid being scammed by someone miss-selling the herbs.

Herbal medicine is not a new phenomenon; it is referred to as traditional medicine and parts of it have slowly been accepted by the medical industry. The Chinese have been using it for years with a lot of success; in fact herbal remedies are referred to as far back as five thousand years ago when the Sumerians recorded a list of plants and the medical uses for each plant. In fact, although a written record exists from five thousand years ago, it is believed that plants were used for healing sixty thousand years ago; this belief is backed by archaeological evidence.

Herbal remedies are often seen as the last resort of patients suffering from cancer, diabetes and asthma. When modern medicine has not managed to resolve an issue then the traditional; herbal medicines are often tried in a bid to improve health or simply slow the spread of a disease. Alkaline herbs are milder and soothing, as well as being more in tune with your body. This makes them a completely natural solution. However; it is important that you seek advice if you are planning on taking herbal remedies; particularly if you are still taking modern medicines as well.

There have been numerous surveys completed into the effectiveness of many different herbs; whilst the results of these indicate that there are none which are truly effective against the more prominent medical conditions. This does not mean it is not worth trying them; you should never give up hope!

Chapter 1 – 5 Alkaline Herbal Remedies for Improved Health

It is a fact of life that your body will be more acidic at key times throughout the day; this can be affected by the food that you eat. Herbal therapists believe it is possible to keep your body more alkaline and less likely to contract specific illnesses. In fact, some people state that alkaline herbs can be beneficial in reducing certain types of cancer or preventing you from getting it. Medical research has not yet managed to prove this theory.

The following five alkaline herbs or herb mixtures are designed to help improve your health and vitality. This is the best possible prevention and care that you can have for your body; a naturally healthy body will be better at fighting off any attack made by germs:

1. *Garlic*

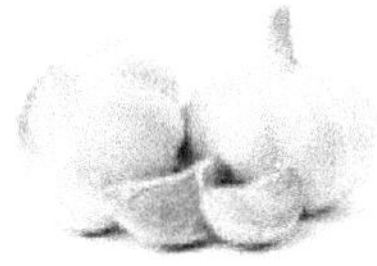

This natural herbal remedy is alkaline in nature and part of the same family as the onion. Although it has a powerful odor and is frequently used in cooking; it also offers a wide range of health benefits. By itself it is an invaluable source of calcium, selenium and phosphorous; as well as an array of important vitamins.

It will help to balance the PH of your system; particularly if you have been consuming a lot of acidic foods. It has also been suggested as offering a range of health benefits, such as lowering blood pressure, reducing coronary problems and even preventing colds and flu. There have even been surveys which suggest it can help to prevent cancer and fight bacterial and fungal infections. It is truly a powerful remedy!

It is worth noting that, if you are not a fan of the smell, then it is possible to consume garlic pills or supplements. These can be purchased as odorless; although this does mean there is a reduced rate of allicin and the supplement is less effective than natural garlic. An alternative is to chew parsley after having garlic is to drink a glass of milk. Both approaches can reduce the taste and after effects of garlic.

2. Dandelions

Most people consider dandelion a weed. However it is a powerful weapon in the herbalist's bag of tricks. In fact, the dandelion leaf can offer an impressive range of health benefits. The most benefit is gained by consuming fresh dandelion leaves which are alkaline and anti-carcinogenic. The dandelion leave has actually been used for many years in salads around the world. It has been shown to help improve your digestion, increase renal activity and even boost your immune system; preventing you from getting those annoying winter colds.

An alternative is to use the roots of the dandelion to produce delicious tea or root beer. Each one has its own unique flavor. Consuming both the root and the leaf will enable your body to stabilize its blood sugar levels; this makes it an invaluable aid for any diabetic.

Perhaps the best thing about dandelion leaves is that they grow anywhere. Although native to the West, they can now be found in India and even parts of the Himalayas. You can grow them in your garden effortlessly, although it is important to plant and pick the right type; there are other plants which bear a striking resemblance. You should also never pick dandelions from the side of the road as they will have been exposed to all kinds of pollutants; any positive health benefits they can offer may be destroyed by the negative effects of these pollutants.

3. Turmeric

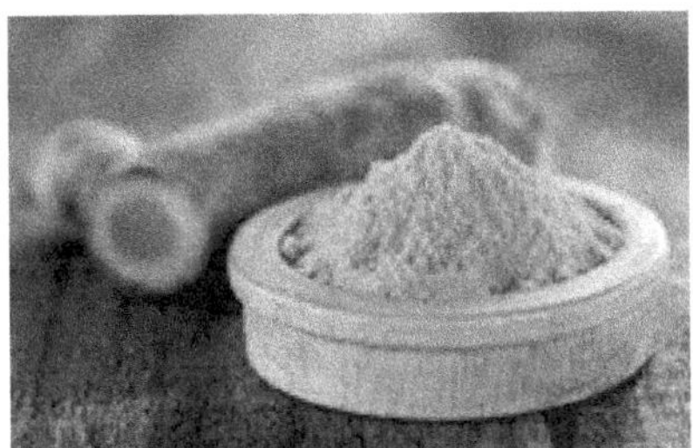

This herb has a real kick. It is often used in the Middle East and adds a spicy flavor to any meal. However, it is more than just an extra bit of flavoring; it is a medicinal herb which can be used for a variety of purposes. In fact, it is potentially one of the most powerful herbs available. It is often referred to as being able to fight disease and even reverse the progress if you are already ill!

Turmeric is known to work better than many over the counter medicines; its list of health benefits includes as an anti-inflammatory, anti-depressant, anti-coagulant and even as a pain killer. Alongside this it is shown to be effective at treating diabetes, arthritis and even reducing cholesterol. As a natural alternative it is safe to be consumed by anyone with an allergy. Of course, the aim is to balance the body and improve your overall health, for this reason it is safest to consult your doctor before you start any treatment. Another benefit of Turmeric is that unless you have an excessive amount of this herb it has been shown to have no real side effects.

4. Lemons

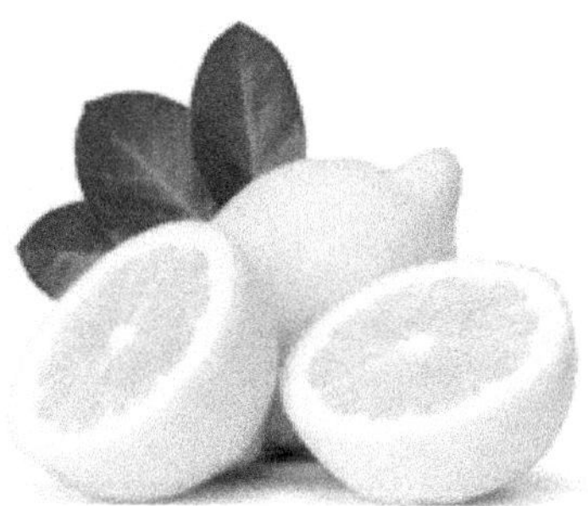

http://dingo.care2.com/pictures/greenliving/1296/1295735.large.jpg

Although technically a fruit, lemons are frequently used by herbalists to help balance the alkaline content of your body. It is often used in cleaning products as a natural cleaning and is even known to have disinfecting properties. Many people have used lemons to detox their bodies and the reason that this is so effective is that lemons are a powerful alkaline and can restore the natural balance of your body.

In fact, lemons can be applied directly to open wounds to help, clean them and heal them. They are also exceptionally effective at providing relief for a variety of viruses; including the common cold and flu. An additional benefit to lemons is the ability to reduce acidity in the body and the cause of heartburn.

Perhaps more importantly as a health benefit a lemon has been shown to revitalize the liver and boost the immune system; contributing to overall health.

5. Chives

This is another herb which can be grown in most gardens. You may already have come across it sprinkled onto salads or as a garnish on other foods. However, you may not have realized that this herb is alkaline reach and has a host of health benefits. It is also possible and easy to add it to almost any meal making it an excellent way to restore the balance in your body.

Chives have been shown to boost your general health and to specifically help the health of your heart. They can also improve your bone strength, help to protect against a range of cancers and give your immune system a much needed boost; effectively protecting against everything. On top of this, regular consumption of chives is believed to improve your eyesight and your digestive system. Finally, they have been shown to be effective when pregnant by preventing birth defects.

The chive is actually another member of the onion family and it is now grown in many places across the world. The edible part of the plant is the slim green shoots which are hollow and add a tasty zing to any meal; whether soup, salad or even a potato dish. Despite being a member of the onion family they do not generally leave the aftertaste, bad breath and general issues which arise from eating onions.

It is useful to know that a chive contains anti-bacteria which are exceptionally effective at combating any gastrointestinal issue. Whilst doing so, it will improve the efficiency and uptake of nutrients from food passing through the intestine; benefitting your body and overall health. The reason it is so good at maintaining bone density is due to the high content of vitamin K found in chives. This vitamin is not found in many food sources making chives an essential part of any diet!

Herbs are a natural and easy way to add nutrients and good bacteria to your body, helping to ensure you remain in good health. This is important, the better balanced your system is the easier you will find it to fight off infections or even prevent them from getting into your body. However, this is only the first stage of what herbs can achieve. As well as helping to maintain your body, they can repair damage and even reverse a variety of illnesses.

Chapter 2 – 5 Alkaline Herbs to reverse Illness

Medical researchers work exceptionally hard every day in an attempt to find cures for the variety of diseases which are in existence. Some of them have split into so many different variations that even finding a cure for one is not enough; it is essential to find something that will treat all the different versions. Cancer is an excellent example of this kind of disease and one that has been around for many years.

Much of the research and medicines which are developed start by using flowers and herbs; these natural products are full of nutrients which are helpful to the human body. Sometimes it is simply a case of locating which herbs to mix together and in what quantities; unfortunately this is a slow and tedious process.

The alternative, especially if there is not a cure created, is to use herbs yourself. They can be added to your food, taken as supplements or even eaten as a snack! If you choose the right herbs you can reverse a range of diseases and improve your overall health.

1. *The Alkaline Diet*

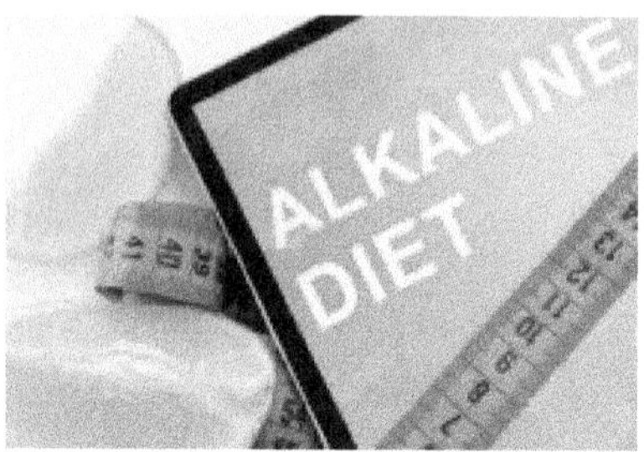

There is a significant amount of research which suggests that an alkaline diet can be beneficial when dealing with cancer, heart disease and even diabetes. In fact, it has even been suggested that this type of diet can help to treat people who have suffered from a stroke, diabetes or even a mental disorder.

The theory behind this diet is that your body is filled with alkaline nutrients and this will boost the phytonutrients in your body which protect against pathogens and toxins. The result is a healthier body which has a reduced level of disease due to the influx of alkaline minerals and an improved immune system to protect against future incidents.

Some of the best herbs to include in this type of life style diet are sarsaparilla and burdock root; although the principle behind this is simply to eat alkaline rich material and leave the acidic food alone. Alongside this change in diet it is recommended that you engage in some exercise as this will boost the blood flow in your body and help to ensure the nutrients and minerals all get to where they need to be.

This diet does not involve just herbs; this would make it very difficult to sustain and be detrimental to your health. However, it does focus on alkaline based foods and herbs to produce some impressive results.

2. Sage

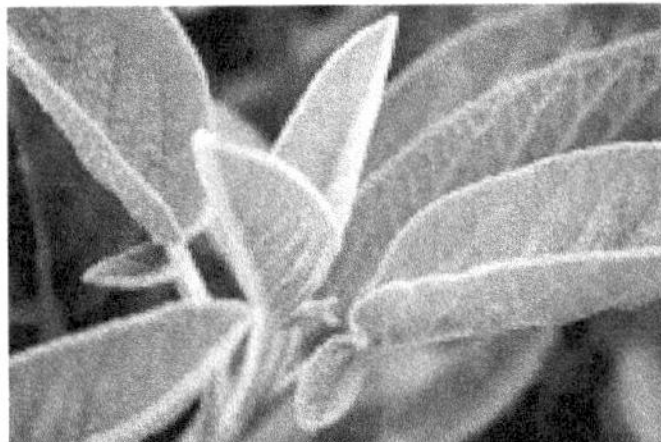

http://static.wixstatic.com/media/ffa001_915d0c47745b4b4baabf0451a6084268.gif

It is a fact of life that you will probably sprain or strain part of your body at some point. This may be the result of a sudden movement or exercise without warming up, or it may be due to an accidental fall. Strains and sprains can be frustrating as they will inhibit your movement and prevent you from undertaking your normal exercise routine. It is important to rest a strain for as long as it needs to get better. In the meantime you can use herbs like sage to help, your injury heal and your body recover. Sage, Thyme and even Rosemary are full of natural oils and flavonoids which have several beneficial effects on your injury.

They act as anti-oxidants and anti-inflammatories. These help to reduce swelling and assist in healing; ensuring that the joint you have strained quickly recovers and allows you to return to your normal routine.

Regular consumption of Sage has also been shown to improve the function of your brain; in particular it is very effective at improving your memory capabilities. You can easily add it to a variety of recipes and improve your overall health.

Sage has also been used by the Chinese for many years. It is known to have a positive effect on anyone suffering from Alzheimer's. In fact, it has been associated with treating cerebrovascular disease since the dawn of the Chinese Empire. The logic behind this treatment is simple but effective. Alzheimer's has been linked to an increase need for AChE which results in the depletion of this chemical from key parts, of the brain. Sage inhibits this depletion and reduces the risk of Alzheimer's and even reverses the condition if it has already started to take hold.

3. Hibiscus Tea

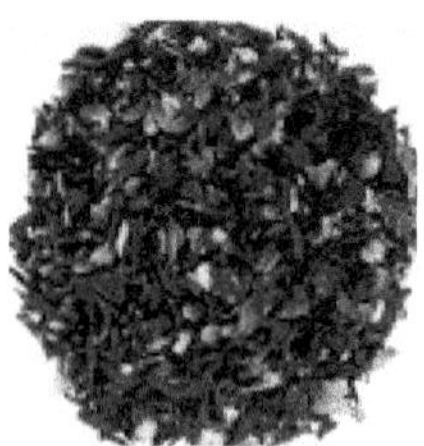

http://to.gstatic.com/images?q=tbn:ANd9GcS7xqJIlrjcgGcyrodsn9jUwRseldZd2NrY39MyHJlc8KnnAZYerD1vRSw

There are a huge number of herbal teas available on the market, almost every flavor and taste bud is accounted for. But herbal teas do more than just smell great; they actually have the power to help improve your health!

Hibiscus tea is made from the Hibiscus plant and has a delicious, fruity flavor. Research into the different types of tea has shown that Hibiscus tea is effective at lowering blood sugar levels and cholesterol. In fact, in animal tests the tea was capable of lowering blood sugar by forty six percent and insulin by fourteen percent. This means that drinking this tea has an immediate health benefit in that it improves your body health. But, it also can help to reverse a variety of diseases, or risk of diseases including coronary disease and diabetes.

4. Tinctures

This is the name given to the extract of herb which has been converted into a liquid and can be taken orally. This is an excellent and easy way to supplement your diet with the benefits of a variety of herbs without the issue of adding herbs to every meal. In one capsule you will receive all the herbs you need.

The capsule is placed under your tongue and will dissolve very quickly. The nutrients are immediately removed from the capsule and go straight into your bloodstream. The liquid is made up of liquid herbs which are either referred to as standard; meaning they have been extracted in alcohol. Or, they can be extracted in apple cider vinegar or even vegetable glycerine.

It is important to remember that a relaxing herb taken this way will have an almost immediate effect which can be very useful if it is an alternative pain relief or relaxant. If the purpose is to build up the nutrients in your body you will find it takes two or three weeks of regular use before the benefits will be visible and show as effective.

The tincture is a small glass tube which has approximately thirty drops of the liquid herb. This is a similar amount to that which you would get in a cup of tea, but, the tincture will supply the herb into your bloodstream much quicker.

It is worth noting that a tincture is a better and more effective way to provide essential nutrients to a child. They may not be interested in sitting and drinking a cup of herbal tea whereas a tincture is fun and takes just a few moments of their time.

5. *Ginger*

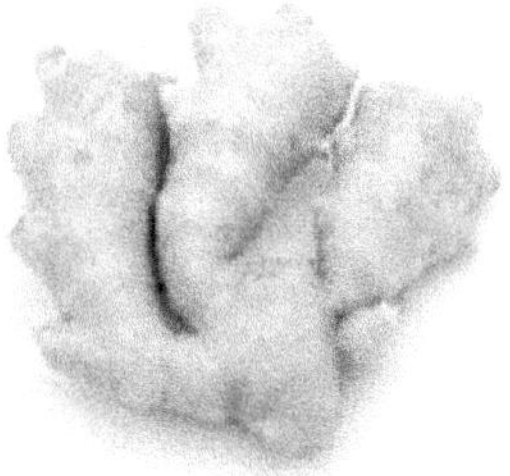

http://t2.gstatic.com/images?q=tbn:ANd9GcSrflryadswssroMNZo_x_eaYSsmQait5i7CHDB9THd0Puzz8TZLUs5cDs

Ginger has been known for many years to have a positive effect on sickness. Whether you are suffering from morning sickness, travel sickness or even just a general nausea you can benefit from taking a little ginger. It has even been known to provide almost instant relief from tooth ache; simply by holding a little piece on the affected tooth.

Ginger actually has a surprisingly low ph rating of approximately 5.6. This is surprising due to the fierce heat it can create in your mouth. It can be added to a variety of food types, meals and even drinks to improve flavor and boost your health.

More importantly there has been extensive research into the effects of ginger on the human body. One which has been shown to justify taking ginger is the reversal of heart disease. This has been linked to a study which suggests that heart disease is often cause by inflammation in the body. Whilst inflammation is important to help the body heal too much of it places a strain on the heart and can result in heart disease. The solution is something as simple as ginger; which has anti-inflammatory properties. Ginger works to reduce inflammation by blocking several genes which cause the inflammation. It is a delicate balance but the ginger will help to prevent the root cause of heart disease and it can be effective even if you already have heart disease!

The easiest and most effective ways to consume ginger is either by adding it to your cooking or by using a little piece of its root to make ginger tea; just allow a piece of ginger to soak in boiling water for half an hour.

Chapter 3 – 5 Ways to Combine the Herbs for the Most effective Results

Herbs can be an additional part of your diet and help you to lead a happier and healthier life. However, the more you read about them the more you will feel you need to consume. This will eventually mean you are spending half your time consuming herbs in a variety of different ways and concoctions. This is unlikely to be a practical way of adding these powerful nutrients into your diet. It is, therefore, essential to work out the most effective way of combining the alkaline herbs and consuming them.

It is essential to remember that these herbs have a powerful effect on your body simply because they are helping to keep its ph level balanced. Although you are unlikely to encounter health problems by having too high an alkaline content in your body the real aim is to keep your body balanced; this will ensure it is in the best possible place to deal with any infection or other issue.

1. Herbs in Food

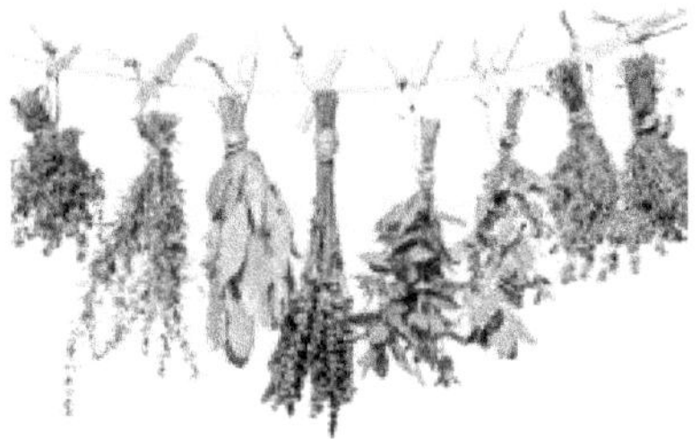

http://t1.gstatic.com/images?q=tbn:ANd9GcTrYgLhlHzUm8Go-cyZ_rhmfyYX141BvC4H1X9XDh6RY9idISgw2hHZ7L4

The most obvious way to get these herbs into your body is through the natural means of consuming them in your food. This is very effective as you can easily prepare the quantity of herbs you wish to consume every day and then add them into your various meals. This will ensure you know how much of any substance you are getting and, if necessary, you can mask the flavor of an herb you believe is beneficial but you do not enjoy the taste of it.

However, it is not as simple as combining all your herbs into one dish and eating them. The human body is a surprisingly delicate machine. The wrong mixture of food can result in heartburn or excess acid, upset stomach or even a serious case of the wind. This is because you have not balanced your food properly. You must consume food which complements each other. This is essential as improper combining will lead to an excess of toxins and potential issues with your digestive system. Part of the equation relates to the types of food you are intending to consume. Some food types simply cannot be broken down by the human body if they are being inhibited by another food type. A key example of this is consuming protein and starch at the same time. Starch needs an alkaline based digestive system for you to completely digest the food and gain the maximum benefits from the nutrients. In contrast the protein your body needs, often found in meat, needs an acid environment to be properly digested. If you eat the two foods at the same time then the acid in your stomach will cancel the alkaline content. In effect you food will simply pass through your body without being properly digested. Not only does this mean that you have failed to get all the nutrients from your food, it also allows undigested food through your body which can cause a variety of issues.

2. Eating Raw Foods

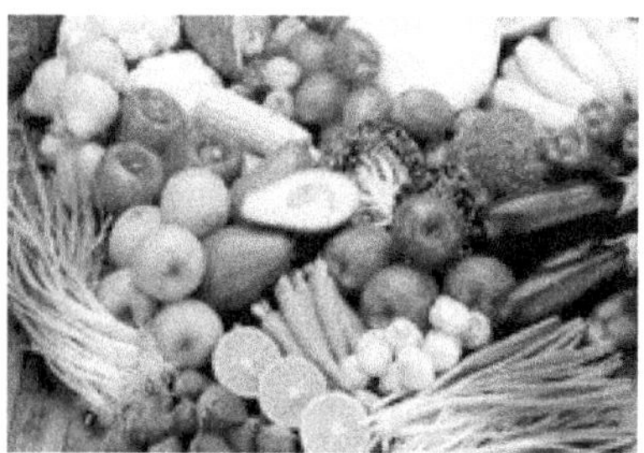

Cooking your food is one way to ensure the nutrients are reduced; it can also help your body to break down the food. However, the issue of combining protein and starch will still remain. An alternative to this is to consume more of your food raw. This is not advocating the consumption of raw meat. However, it is worth considering the basis of humanity. The human body was initially designed to eat raw fruit and vegetables, particularly leafy greens and fruit. This was the diet for many people in ancient times, before hunting and food processing took over. The advantage of greens and fruit is that they are generally happy being digested in a neutral environment; not too acidic or alkaline. Although this type of food is generally full of nutrients and other valuable minerals, it is easy to digest and passes through your body with minimal resistance; ensuring your gut stays healthy and there are no difficult to digest pieces which block up your system and create bloating or wind. (These are two of the biggest signs that you have a digestive issue).

It has also been suggested that this type of diet places less stress on the digestive system and, therefore, saves your energy to allow you to use it on other things.

3. Supplements

One of the easiest ways to get any vitamin or nutrient into your body is via a supplement. There are many different herbal supplements which can be found in your local health store. However, it is important to note that not all supplements will provide as much benefit as eating the herbs. You will also still need to eat and be faced with the problem of what to eat and how best to combine your food to get the right results, both for your ongoing health and to reduce any diseases you already have.

It is essential to consider carefully which supplements you are planning to mix, although you may only be taking a pill the nutrients you will be adding into your body can conflict with each other and with any prescription drugs you are taking; although you are probably trying to reduce your support on prescription drugs. A further consideration which may affect your decision to take supplements is that not all herbal based supplements are approved; the legislation on this type of product does not specify the requirement for a review. It is therefore possible that you are purchasing a supplement which is not what it says it is. You should ensure any herbal supplements you purchase are bought from a reputable source.

4. *Know your herb*

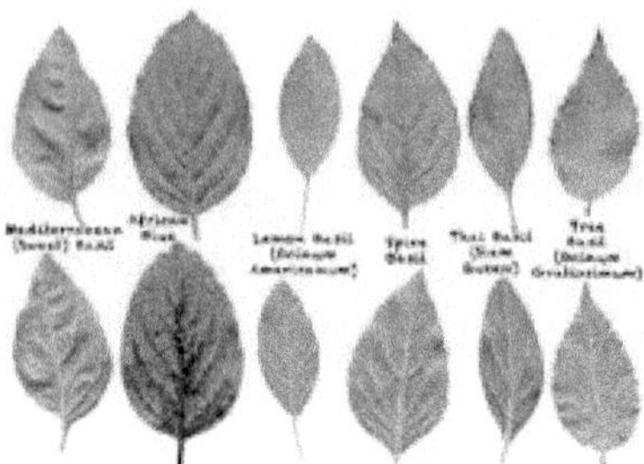

If you are harvesting your own herbs it is essential that you know which herb is which. There are many incidents in nature where two plants can be physically very similar but have very different qualities. Before you eat anything you must be certain it is what you think it is.

It is also essential to consider the way you prepare the herb. Eating the leaves will introduce the nutrients into your body in a different way to brewing a tea or crushing the root. You must be certain that you know what your intended result is and the right way to get that result. You will also find that taking two herbs with similar properties are likely to cancel each other out; leaving you with no discernable benefit.

A final point to be wary of if you have not taken a specific herb before is your health. Even if the herb is supposed to help you recover from a disease, you do not know if you will have a reaction to it. You should always check with a small amount first.

5. *Learn Your Diet*

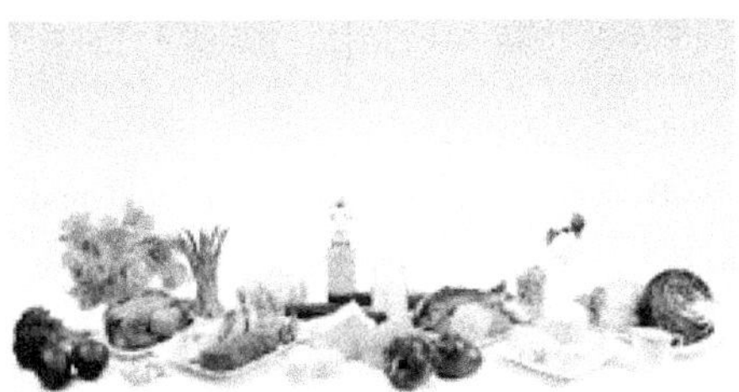

http://t3.gstatic.com/images?q=tbn:ANd9GcSomlAGUWOxSGjWF7ZxMtUozKOIf_oDxUN-uKpZeork5AuZEp2X_d-Ex2Do

Point one of this chapter touched on the importance of not combining proteins and starch as your body will not be able to digest it properly. To help understand this concept a little further the following guide will help you know what to eat with what:

Leafy Green can be processed fairly easily by your body and are acceptable to accompany most meals.

Other vegetables tend to be harder to digest and will have starch in them. You should avoid eating these with fruit. Instead put them with protein, such as meat.

Beans are generally cooked before eating and will then break down easier in your body; although it is rare for them to break down completely. You can combine them with other vegetables.

Starch is present in potatoes, wheat, bread and pasta; amongst other things. They should be combined with the leafy greens but never with protein.

 Protein takes the most effort for your body to breakdown and needs an acid environment. You should combine protein rich food with leafy greens and avoid eating too much of them. There is little you can combine protein with; you may have to just wait until it has been digested. Once you have gained an understanding of how the body digests different types of food you will be able to adjust your eating habits to maximize the benefit to your body.

Conclusion

Despite the abundance of diets and exercise regimes very few people consider the impact of what you eat and how it affects your body's ability to do certain things. Even more importantly, many aches, pains and other uncomfortable sensations can be eliminated simply by looking at the way your body processes food.

This book is designed to teach you which herbs are alkaline and can help you stay healthy; but it is also intended to show you that the best way of staying healthy is to respect your body's natural limits. Simple science shows that something which dissolves in acid will not dissolve in an alkaline; yet you are asking your body to perform this all the time! Learning which foods to combine and which should be eaten separately will allow you to maximize the nutrition from the food you eat and will ensure your body digests it properly. Foods which dissolve in alkaline mixtures will also dissolve in an acid; however, you will not gain the same level of benefit from these foods as the acid will destroy much of the goodness. This is why it is essential to understand which foods can be mixed and which should be eaten separately.

Many people who adopt this style of eating will drift towards a more fruit or vegan based diet, but this does not have to be the case. Meat is acceptable; providing it is not eaten at the same time as starch. This is perhaps the most important lesson to understand as it goes against the principles of eating in the western world where meat, potatoes and vegetables are the norm.

Alkaline herbs and the combination of foods you eat will make it possible for you to enjoy a healthy life without many of the pains that most people suffer from, such as bloating and trapped wind. This is a product of western diets and one that can be avoided with a little education and a little extra thought about the foods you eat.

It should be noted that you do not need to switch to an alkaline diet, but you must become more aware of the effect of acids and alkaline foods on your digestive system. Mixing the two is never desirable and places considerable strain on your body. Once you start watching what you are eating and combining foods properly you will quickly realize that it is easy to stick to this type of eating patterns. But, what you will notice is that you will no longer be able or even want to eat the majority of processed foods which do mix proteins and starches; they are generally designed for convenience as opposed to health.

FREE Bonus Reminder

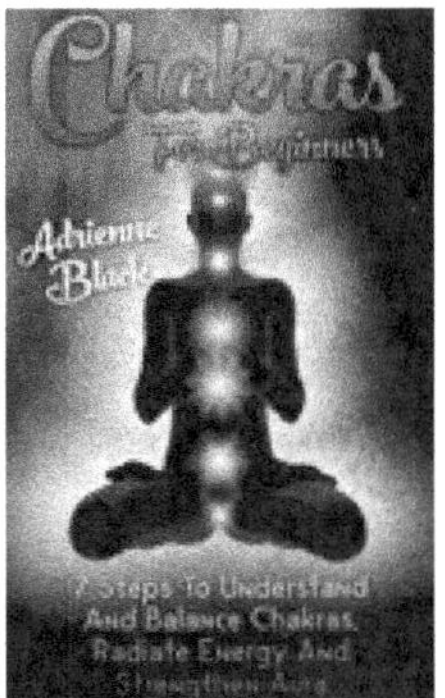

If you have not grabbed it yet, please go ahead and download your special bonus E book *"Chakras for Beginners. 7 Steps To Understand And Balance Chakras, Radiate Energy, And Strengthen Aura"*.

Simply Click the Button Below

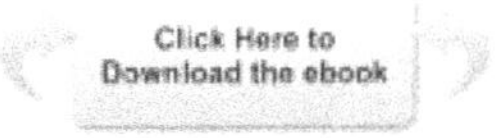

OR Go to This Page

http://lifehacksworld.com/free

BONUS #2: More Free & Discounted Books & Products

Do you want to receive more Free/Discounted Books or Products?

We have a mailing list where we send out our new Books or Products when they go free or with a discount on Amazon. Click on the link below to sign up for Free & Discount Book & Product Promotions.

=> Sign Up for Free & Discount Book & Product Promotions <=

OR Go to this URL

http://zbit.ly/1WBb1Ek